BEGINNER'S GUIDE TO

MEATLESS CASSEROLES

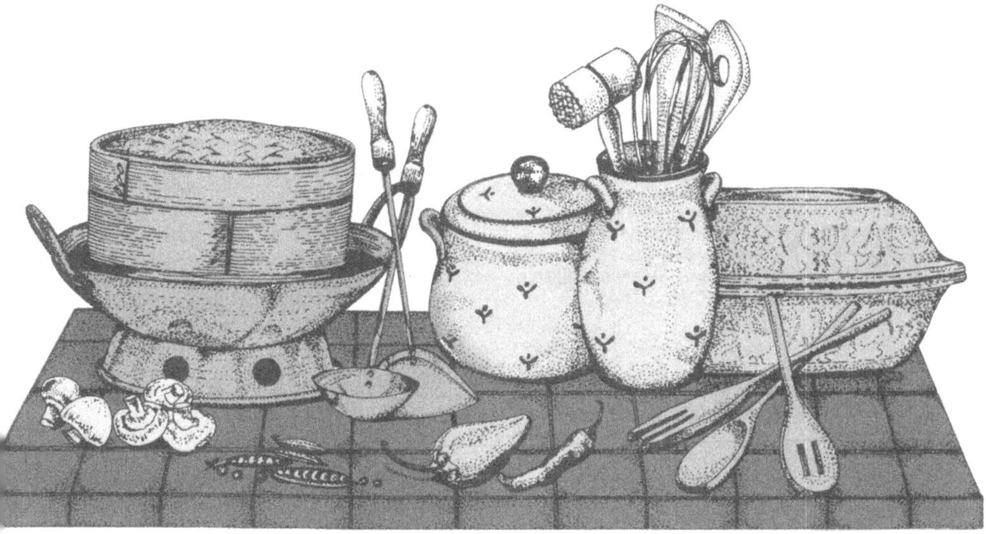

by Ellen Sue Spicer-Jacobson - revised and expanded edition

Beginner's Guide to Meatless Casseroles

This revised edition of the *Beginner's Guide to Meatless Casseroles* would not have been possible without the encouragement of my assistant Lynn Allopenna, the faith of my editor Franz Ross, and the truthful responses from my "test panel"—my family and friends. Thanks also go to Nancy Cleaver and Linda Cook for their terrific graphics.

Published by:
Ross Books
P.O. Box 4340
Berkeley, Calif. 94704
ISBN 978-0-89496-039-0
web: www.rossbooks.com

Preface to the Second Edition

When I first compiled these recipes in 1975, I was a novice vegetarian. Almost all of my dishes were made with eggs or dairy products, and I relied heavily on the theory of complementary proteins. Since then, I have realized that protein is virtually in everything we eat. I now often make wholesome meatless dishes without dairy or eggs, and I rely on nuts, tofu, and tahini for obvious protein sources.

With regard to *all* ingredients, I recommend using *whole* grain noodles, *fresh* fruits and vegetables, and *sprouted* grains and beans. Also, if you intend to use cheese, use only natural cheese, not cheese-food or processed cheese. Whenever possible, purchase preservative-free and chemical-free products; choose grains and produce from organic farms. Quality is the important word.

Raw foods now occupy a more prominent place in my diet. Sun-ripened, uncooked foods retain more of the enzymes and nutrients with which Mother Nature intended to nourish us. At our home, meals of any kind are always served behind a large, fresh salad and a fresh, steamed or stir-fried vegetable. Often our "main dish" *is* the salad and vegetables. Casseroles, however, are an excellent way to move into meatless meals since meat is not always necessary to complete a dish.

This revised edition, then, is broken down into three categories: noodles; potatoes; grains and beans. For each recipe I have included utensils and tips as well as a few serving suggestions to help you plan your menu. A glossary has been provided to define terms that may be unfamiliar to you.

I have also given you more flexibility with each recipe. In the first edition, for example, I listed oil as the only medium for sauteing vegetables. Recent literature has pointed out that oil heated to high temperatures is not healthy. I have experimented with broths, vegetable juices, and just plain water. When the recipe lists all these, choose whichever you prefer. When listing dry herbs and spices, I prefer to leave the amount and type up to you. If you use fresh herbs, remember to double the amount.

I no longer use refined table salt with my meals. If you still want salt, try natural soy sauce or Miso-Cup™ (a soybean product that can be used as a condiment or made into a broth.) Likewise, Sprinkle™ and Nature's Gourmet™ are two salt-free products that I highly recommend. Our own company (Deep Roots) has developed a tasty salt alternative: Whole Herb Seasoning. It contains parsley, garlic, thyme, sage, marjoram, and freeze-dried alfalfa sprouts. It's a seasoning for almost any dish. If you cannot find it at your supermarket, our friends at Walnut Acres, Penns Creek, PA 17862, will mail you a jar. Send for their free catalog.

Finally, in this second edition I omitted Miscellaneous Dishes with Sprouts because I am publishing a more comprehensive *Beginner's Guide to Meals with Sprouts*. Watch for it.

Additionally, in each recipe, the ingredients have been aligned with the directions enabling quick and easy reference during the cooking process.

Thinking I have made mention of all the new additions, I find two more emphatics to let loose: *don't* be afraid to experiment and *do* be creative. Cooking is just as much an art as it is a skill. Go to it.

Preface to the First Edition

My decision to eat less meat was a gradual one. Luckily for me, two great vegetarian cookbooks were already in print: *Diet for a Small Planet* by Frances Moore Lappe' and *Recipes for a Small Planet* by Ellen Buchman Ewald. They helped *me* get started.

Later, I began to teach meatless cooking, passing on my newly gained knowledge of meatless meals to others. As we cooked casseroles and main dishes each week, I realized that all the students were beginners in the area of meatless cooking. I then developed some simplified recipes to help beginners get started with confidence. This booklet is for those of you who would like to try cooking more meals without meat but are having difficulty getting in gear.

One great advantage of these recipes is that many of them can be prepared in advance and popped in the oven or left simmering on the stove an hour or less before dinner. Also, if you double the recipe, you can serve half and freeze the uncooked half for a future meal.

In order to obtain maximum nutrition from these dishes, start with basic, unrefined ingredients such as beans, seeds, nuts, brown rice, honey, cheese, yogurt, etc., at your supermarket or at a health food store. With these basic items on hand, along with some fresh vegetables and fruits, you can put together a tasty, nutritious, meatless dish. Whenever possible, use foods in their raw state. For example, garnish a casserole with slivers of raw food. Serve a raw salad or a single raw food with the cooked dish.

Second, to retain more of the valuable nutrients from your fresh vegetables and grains, I recommend that you:

1. Save the water from cooked beans and use it again for soups, gravies, and other recipes calling for stock.

2. Steam fresh vegetables over water instead of cooking *in* the water. If you don't own a vegetable steamer, use a colander that fits inside a pot with a tight lid. Use only a couple inches of water to steam your vegetables for a few minutes. You should also consider purchasing a *wok* (a Chinese cooking pot which stir-fries the food quickly and with very little loss of food value). A pressure cooker is also handy for preparing basic ingredients quickly.

A final word of CAUTION: Start with dishes that are similar to what you may already like or are accustomed to. Or serve a new dish first "on the side," and gradually use it as a main dish. Little by little, you will begin to enjoy many of these different flavors and new food tastes. Don't be discouraged if a dish doesn't "go over well." Keep trying and make substitutions if necessary. The variety is endless. Remember to go slowly at first, and soon, your meatless dishes will become an integral part of your meals.

Contents

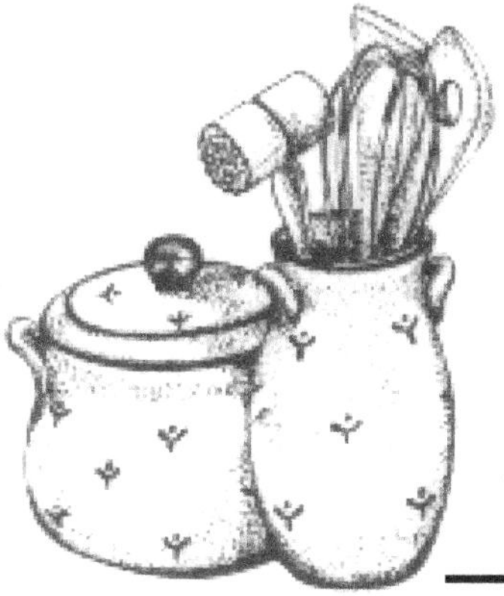

NOODLES

I suggest using whole wheat or whole grain noodles in these recipes. Whole grain noodles, which come in a variety of shapes and shades, are made with the entire kernel or grain and therefore contain more of the natural, wholesome ingredients. If you have never eaten whole grain noodles, however, I recommend that you first try the recipes with the noodles you normally use and then gradually add the whole grain noodles in successive recipes.

There are also wide varieties of pasta flours from which to choose: Jerusalem artichoke noodles, which look like traditional white noodles but which are made from a combination of soy flour and artichoke flour; all whole wheat noodles; all corn noodles; whole wheat and sesame; sesame and soy; and spinach or buckwheat noodles in a base of whole wheat. For instructions on how to cook noodles, see Cooking Hints.

Special Spaghetti Sauce

This sauce recipe can be used in any of the recipes calling for tomato sauce.

Ingredients

1. Olive oil, butter or tomato juice
1-2 garlic cloves, peeled and minced
1 onion, peeled and chopped

2. 1-2 bell peppers, minced
6-8 mushrooms, washed and sliced
1 small eggplant, washed and sliced
8 cups tomato sauce

3. Spices: oregano, basil and thyme

Directions

1. Saute the garlic and onion in a large sauce pan or dutch oven, using oil, butter or juice.

2. When the onions are soft, add peppers, mushrooms, and eggplant. Pour into tomato sauce.

3. Add the spices and simmer them with the lid slightly ajar, until the eggplant is tender and saturated with the sauce (about 1 hour).

Spaghetti Dorio

This dish is a nice alternative to the traditional spaghetti with tomato sauce. It is colorful, tasty, and can be quickly prepared.

Utensils

Measuring Cup
Frying pan for vegetables
Cutting board and knife
Large cooking pot for noodles
Colander
Grater (If you are using cheese)
Attractive serving bowl (optional)

Ingredients

1. 1-2 garlic cloves, peeled and minced
1 onion, peeled and chopped
Oil, butter, or stock

2. 1 cup minced vegetables in season (e.g., eggplant, pepper, yellow squash, and zucchini)
Water
Spices to taste: oregano, basil, and thyme

3. 1 lb. thin spaghetti or fettucini noodles, preferably whole grain
$^1/_4$ cup sesame or olive oil
$^2/_3$ cup sesame seeds (toasted or un-toasted)
1 cup grated natural cheese (optional)

Directions

1. In a frying pan, saute the garlic and onion in a small amount of oil until they are soft. (This takes less than 5 minutes.)

2. Add the minced vegetables and small amount of water. Cover and simmer until vegetables are tender, but not mushy. (This takes less than 15 minutes.)

During the last few minutes, stir in the spices for tasting purposes. Hint: You should now start boiling the water for the noodles.

Remove the cooked vegetables from the stove and keep them covered.

3. While the vegetables are simmering, cook the noodles in a large pot according to the directions on the package.

Drain the noodles and replace them in the same pot without the water. Toss with oil, seeds, and cooked vegetables. If you are using cheese, sprinkle it on the noodles and toss them again gently.

Transfer to an attractive serving bowl and serve at once.

Tips

Since the preparation time Is only a little longer than the time for cooking noodles, have the table set and the salad ready to eat.

Grate the cheese while the noodles and vegetables are cooking.

Spinach Spaghetti and Seeds

Although this is a simple version of Spaghetti Dorio, it is too good just to be considered a variation.

Utensils

Measuring Cup
Large pot for noodles
Blender or Jar
Colander
Grater (If you ore using cheese)
Attractive serving bowl (optional)

Ingredients

1. $^1/_4$ cup sesame, olive, or safflower oil
1-2 garlic cloves, peeled and minced (or use dehydrated garlic) and oregano, basil and thyme

2. 1 Ib. spinach spaghetti or spinach ribbons
1 cup mixed seeds: sesame, poppy and caraway (or dill)

Directions

1. Put the ingredients in a blender and buzz or place in a jar and shake well.
Set aside.

2. Cook the noodles according to package directions. Drain and place them back in the pot without any water.

Toss them with oil mixture and seeds (and cheese if you are using it). Transfer to an attractive serving bowl and serve at once.

Tips

This dish requires even less cooking time than Spaghetti Dorio; so hove your dinner ready to eat.

Pre-mix oil and spices; pre-mix seeds.

Grate cheese before starting the noodles.

Quick 'n' Easy Noodles with Eggplant

This one-dish meal takes very little time to prepare, especially if you have leftover noodles.

Utensils

Large frying pan or dutch oven for eggplant
Measuring cup
Large pot for noodles
Grater for cheese
Heatproof casserole dish (optional)

Ingredients

1. Tomato juice or thin tomato sauce
3-4 chopped scallions
1 garlic clove, peeled and minced
1 small eggplant, washed and diced (with or without skins)

2. 3 cups whole grain noodles, any shape, or 8 oz. spaghetti
2 cups seasoned tomato sauce

3. $1^1/_2$ - 2 cups grated natural cheese
2-3 T. sesame seeds (raw or toasted)

Directions

1. In a large pan or dutch oven, saute scallions, garlic, and eggplant in a small amount of juice, adding water if necessary to prevent sticking. After five minutes, reduce heat to low, cover, and cook for about 10-15 minutes more.

2. Boil the noodles while the eggplant is cooking. When the noodles are done, drain them and then stir them into the pan along with the eggplant.

Pour in the seasoned sauce and simmer 5-10 minutes, or until the eggplant is tender.

3. Add grated cheese to the eggplant and noodles. Sprinkle on the seeds.
Simmer just until the cheese melts.

Tips

Boil water for the noodles and grate the cheese while the eggplant is cooking.

Variation

Transfer the noodles and eggplant to a heatproof, oiled casserole. Add cheese and seeds and bake uncovered until the cheese melts. Use a 300-350° oven.

Garden Vegetables Over Noodles

Utensils

Fry pan or dutch oven for vegetables
Large pot for noodles
9" x 12" heatproof casserole dish or roasting pan
Cutting board and knife
Measuring cup
Colander
Grater

Ingredients

1. Small amount of butter, sesame oil, or stock
1 garlic clove, peeled and minced
1 onion, peeled and chopped

2. 5 cups (approximately) cleaned and minced vegetables, e.g.
1 yellow squash, 1 zucchini, 1 bell pepper, 1 small eggplant
1 cup tomato juice, water, or stock
Herbs and spices to taste; oregano, thyme, natural soy sauce

3. 12—16 oz. whole wheat ribbon noodles
3½ quarts boiling water
1½ cups grated natural cheese (e.g. longhorn)
2 T. sesame seeds, raw or roasted
Lecithin and safflower oil for casserole

Directions

1. In a large frying pan or dutch oven, saute the garlic and onion in a small amount of butter, sesame oil or stock for 2-3 minutes.

2. Add minced vegetables and 1 cup of liquid to the onion and garlic.
Cover and simmer this until the vegetables are tender but not mushy (about 15 minutes).

Add the herbs and spices during the last few minutes. (Start boiling water for the noodles during this time.)

3. While the vegetables are simmering, cook the noodles according to package directions.

Drain and spoon into an oiled casserole. Add the vegetables and the remaining liquid, sprinkle cheese and seeds on, and bake in 350° oven just until cheese melts.

Tips

Oil the casserole before you start to cook. I prefer a combination of liquid lecithin and safflower oil for a goof-proof non-stick surface.

Turn oven on to 350° when the noodles and vegetables are almost done.

Lynn's Luscious Lasagne

This vegetarian lasagna was prepared by my first assistant, Lynn, whose love of pasta is a family tradition.

Utensils

Measuring cup
Large sauce pan for sauce
Large pot for noodles
Potato masher
Ladle
8" x 12" lasagna pan (rectangular deep pan)
Grater for cheese

Ingredients

1. 1 Ib. whole wheat or lasagna-style Jerusalem artichoke noodles*

2. 2 lbs. well-drained tofu or ricotta cheese, or a mixture of the two

3. 2 qts. spaghetti sauce (see sauce recipe)
$^1/_2$ - 1 lb. grated mozzarella cheese or one of your choice

Directions

1. While the sauce is simmering, cook the lasagna noodles according to package directions. Drain and submerge them in cold water to prevent sticking.

2. Mash the drained tofu with a fork or potato masher and then set the tofu aside. (Add spices if you wish.)

3. Using the lasagna pan, make a thick layer of sauce. Add one layer of drained noodles, one layer of sauce, one layer of tofu, and one layer of cheese. Repeat until the top layer ends with noodles, sauce and grated cheese.

Bake in 350° oven until the cheese melts and the dish is heated through.

Tips

Drain and mash tofu and set It aside.
Keep the drained noodles in pan of cool water while assembling the dish.

Variation

Add some minced spinach to the tofu.

*These look like white noodles, but are less starchy and made with soy flour and Jerusalem artichoke flour.

Shells and Cheese

This is a variation on the old stand-by, macaroni and cheese. You can experiment with different noodles and different vegetables of your choice.

Utensils

Roasting pan or large casserole dish (lasagne size pan works well)
Large saucepan for noodles
Large bowl
Cutting board and knife
Grater for cheese and carrots
Blender

Ingredients

1. 6 cups (1 lb.) small shell noodles or vegetable elbow macaroni (whole wheat or mixed grains)

2. 2 medium zucchini, peeled and chopped
2 small onions, peeled and chopped
1 cup water or stock

3. 1 carrot, grated

4. 2 cups grated natural cheese (try mixing two kinds)
Spices to taste: oregano, basil, parsley.

5. $^{1}/_{2}$ - 1 cup (additional) grated cheese
1-2 T. sesame seeds
Sprinkle of paprika
Alfalfa sprouts (optional)

Directions

1. Cook the shells according to the package directions. Drain and place them in a large bowl with pureed vegetables (step 2).

2. While the noodles are cooking, puree the zucchini and onions with water or stock in a blender.
Pour into large bowl and mix gently with cooked noodles.

3. Add the grated carrot to the bowl of noodles and vegetables.

4. Finally, add the 2 cups grated cheese and spices, mixing to distribute evenly.

Place all in the oiled casserole and bake in a 350° oven for about 30 minutes, or until crust begins to form.

5. During the last 10 minutes, remove the casserole, sprinkle on additional cheese, seeds, and paprika, and bake for another 10-15 minutes. (When serving, garnish with fresh alfalfa sprouts for color and crunch.)

Tips

Oil the casserole before you start to cook.

Prepare the vegetables and cheese while the noodles are cooking so that the whole dish can be assembled once the noodles are drained.

Pasta/Bean Bake

This hearty dish can be made with any bean of your choice and any shape noodle you prefer, except perhaps thin spaghetti. It is filling, nutritious, low costing, and tasty.

Utensils

Large pot for vegetables and beans
Large pot for cooking noodles
Cutting board and knife
Colander
Measuring cup
Grater (if you are using cheese)

Ingredients

1. 1-2 carrots, scrubbed and thinly sliced
   1-2 celery stalks, scrubbed and chopped
   1 onion, peeled and diced
   1 garlic clove, peeled and minced
   Tomato juice or sauce or stock

2. 1 cup (dry) navy beans, soaked overnight, drained and frozen on a cookie sheet
   3 cups water or stock

3. 2-3 cups whole wheat elbow noodles or shells
   3 qts. water (boiled)

4. 3 cups tomato sauce
   Spices and herbs to taste: oregano, dill, thyme
   1 cup grated natural cheese (optional)

Directions

1. Simmer the vegetables in a small amount of liquid for about 10 minutes in large pot.

2. Add the frozen beans to the vegetables, adding water or stock, and cook for another 35 minutes, or until beans are tender to taste.

3. Ten to 15 minutes before the beans are done, start the noodles. Cook according to package directions. Drain them and add to the cooked beans.

4. Add tomato sauce and herbs and simmer for 5-10 minutes to allow the flavors to mingle.

If you wish, stir in the cheese during the last 5-10 minutes. Serve warm.

Tips

Cook the noodles offer you hove cut the vegetables so that the warm pasta can be added to the beans, and then the dish can be served almost Immediately.

When reheating, additional liquid may be necessary.

Chilled Pasta Plotter

This dish lends itself to leftover noodles and is perfect for summer lunches.

Utensils

Large pot for noodles
Grater
Blender

Ingredients

1. 16 oz. spinach spaghetti or other whole grain noodle

2. 1 cup olive oil
2 T. mixed herbs: garlic, oregano, basil
2 T. seeds: poppy, sesame, caraway or dill

3. 2 carrots, scrubbed and grated
5-6 radishes, scrubbed and grated
5-6 scallions, cleaned, trimmed, and minced

4. 2 cups whole wheat croutons or 1 cup grated cheese

Directions

1. Cook noodles according to package directions, but rinse with cold water, drain, and chill.

2. Buzz oil and herbs in a blender, add seeds by hand and refrigerate dressing in a closed jar for a few hours.

3. Toss the vegetables with the chilled spaghetti. Add this to the dressing and toss again.

4. Sprinkle on croutons or grated cheese and serve.

Tips

Cook the noodles the night before you intend to make this dish. Rinse them with cold water, drain, and store covered.

Prepare the dressing and chill it a few hours before the meal.

Noodles and Kasha Casserole

This casserole is a meatless version of a traditional Eastern European dish. Roasted buckwheat grits, better known as kasha, are found in most supermarkets, although whole groats might be easier to purchase in a natural foods store.

Utensils

Measuring cup
Large pot for noodles
Roasting pan for kasha
Small fry pan for vegetables
Cutting board and knife
Colander
Heatproof serving dish (optional)

Ingredients

1. 12-16 oz. whole grain noodles, such as spirals or shells
Sesame oil or butter
$^1/_4$ - $^1/_2$ cup sesame seeds, roasted or raw

2. 1 cup (whole) roasted buckwheat groats, rinsed and drained
2 cups boiling water or stock

3. 1 onion, peeled and sliced thin
1 garlic clove, peeled and minced
1 cup mushrooms, washed and sliced (optional)
Oil, butter, or stock
Herbs and spices to taste: parsley flakes, thyme, marjoram

Directions

1. Cook the noodles according to package directions. Drain and toss them with oil or butter (more or less to your taste) and seeds.

2. Set this aside until the kasha is cooked.
Spread the rinsed groats thinly onto a roasting pan and roast them until the grains are dry (about 5-7 minutes), stirring often.
Pour in the boiling liquid, stir, cover, and bake another 15-20 minutes, or until all liquid is absorbed. Uncover during last few minutes. (If you are using buckwheat grits instead of whole groats, the cooking time will be less.)

3. While the noodles and kasha are cooking, saute the onion, garlic, and mushrooms in oil, butter or broth until the vegetables are soft, adding herbs and spices near the end of cooking.
When soft, stir onion, garlic, mushrooms and seasonings into the cooked kasha. Then mix in the cooked noodles (which are already mixed with oil and seeds). Bake for another couple of minutes to heat the entire dish.
Serve from the roasting pan or transfer to an attractive serving dish. Dot with butter or mix with a little oil and serve.

Tips

You should start boiling the water for both kasha and noodles while you are assembling the ingredients.
Preheat oven to 350°F.
Lightly oil a casserole dish if you plan to use one.

Variation

In place of or in addition to the noodles, add steamed peas, carrots,
cauliflower, or broccoli pieces to the cooked kasha.

Confetti Macaroni Casserole

This chilled noodle dish makes an attractive "covered dish" for picnics and gatherings or an interesting whole meal salad for lunch.

Utensils

Measuring cup
Saucepan for eggs
Saucepan for noodles
Cutting board and knife
Blender or hand egg beater
Attractive serving bowl

Ingredients

1. 5 hard-boiled eggs or try cubes of drained tofu (optional)

2. 1 lb. whole wheat or mixed grain elbow macaroni

3. Tofunnaise or your favorite natural mayonnaise

4. $^1/_3$ cup each (washed well):
   diced radishes
   chopped celery
   grated carrot
   diced bell pepper
   minced scallions

5. $^1/_2$ cup raw, unsalted hulled sunflower seeds. (Roast for crunchier taste.)

Directions

1. Boil the eggs for 10-15 minutes. Peel while they are warm. Keep them covered while they are being chilled. (This dish is good even without eggs.) If using tofu, cube or dice.

2. Cook the noodles according to package directions. Drain, rinse, and chill.

3. Prepare the dressing and refrigerate.

4. If you are using eggs, chop the chilled eggs and place them in a bowl with the chilled noodles and dressing. If using diced tofu, stir in gently with vegetables. Gently fold in the cut vegetables.

5. Spoon the noodle mixture into an attractive serving bowl, sprinkle on seeds and serve, or cover and refrigerate until serving time.

Tips

Cook the noodles and eggs, and prepare the dressing early in the day or the night before you prepare this dish, and keep refrigerated until the dish is to be assembled. Drain tofu and wrap in towel and press between two plates with pot on top as a weight.

Tofunnoise

Ingredients

1. $^1/_4$ A cup water
1 T. vegetable oil
Juice of $^1/_2$ lemon
$^1/_2$ t. natural soy sauce
4 oz. firm tofu, drained
$^1/_2$ t. turmeric for color (optional)

Directions

1. Place all ingredients in a blender in the order given. Puree until smooth. Yields about $^1/_4$ cup.

Note: Dressing tends to thicken upon refrigeration. If used the following day, additional water may need to be added.

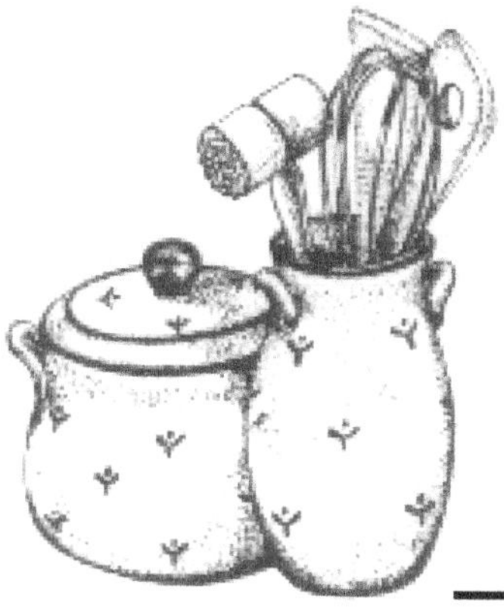

POTATOES

Potatoes are a good food investment nutritionally as well as financially. Besides being one of the least expensive vegetables, white potatoes are high in Vitamin C, iron, potassium, and some B-vitamins. Moreover, a medium-sized white potato boiled in the skin contains only 21 carbohydrate grams (about 90 calories). One medium sized raw apple contains 18 grams and one medium-sized banana has 33.3 grams.

Sweet potatoes contain high levels of Vitamin A and Vitamin C, and fair amounts of calcium, phosphorous, magnesium and natural sodium. One medium cooked sweet potato has 141 calories.

Don't shy away from these few potato recipes because you are afraid they are too fattening. All potato calories are slow-burning, complex carbohydrates rather than simple sugars. The nutrient sum is worth the calorie investment. If you keep away from sour cream toppings, eat normal portions, and consider keeping the skins on the potato for extra nutrition, you're on your way. (Use red-skinned "new" potatoes for added color.)

Potato Vegetable Pie

This inexpensive dish is colorful and tasty, and lends itself to sweet potatoes and white potatoes. It is a potato lover's delight.

Utensils

8"-9" pie plate
Small fry pan for vegetables
Cutting board and knife
Grater (If cheese will be used)

Ingredients

1. 1 lb. sweet potatoes (about 3 medium)
Small amount of oil or butter
Lecithin and safflower oil for pie plate

2. 3-4 scallions, cleaned and chopped
$^1/_2$ - 1 bell pepper, chopped
1-2 celery stalks, scrubbed and chopped
4-5 small mushrooms, chopped
$^1/_2$ small yellow squash, minced
Oil, butter, or stock
Herbs and spices to taste: parsley, garlic, thyme

3. $^1/_2$ - 1 cup grated natural cheese (optional)
2 T. sesame seeds, raw or roasted

Directions

1. Bake or steam the potatoes until they are soft. Peel and mash them with a small amount of oil or butter and press them lightly into a slightly greased pie plate (including the oiled rim).

2. While the potatoes are cooking, simmer the vegetables in a covered frying pan in a small amount of butter, oil or stock until vegetables are soft—but not mushy—for about 10-15 minutes.

Add the seasonings at the end.

Spoon the cooked vegetables into an oiled pie plate lined with the mashed potatoes.

3. Sprinkle the cheese on if you are using it and top with seeds.

Bake in 350°F. oven until the cheese melts or until the potato forms a light crust.

Note: When serving, this dish does not come out as a wedge of pie but rather as a casserole.

Tips

Bake a large batch of sweet potatoes one night for dinner. Use any leftovers for potato pie crust. If you do pre-bake the potatoes, you may wish to steam them for 5 minutes when making the pie so mashing will be easier.

Sliced Potato-Cheese Bake

Since all the ingredients in this dish are assembled raw*, once put together, just pop in the oven and you're finished!

Utensils

Cutting board and knife
Grater for cheese
Oblong baking dish

Ingredients

1. Safflower oil and liquid lecithin

2. 3 large potatoes, scrubbed and sliced thinly
1 cup grated natural cheese (try mixing two kinds)
1 small onion, peeled and chopped
Herbs and spices to taste: thyme, rosemary, chives

3. $^1/_3$ cup milk (raw, if possible) or stock
$^1/_2$ cup caraway seeds or dill seeds

Directions

1. Spread the oils onto an oblong baking dish. (I use wax paper for this and then discard it.)

2. Place a single layer of sliced potatoes on the bottom of the oiled baking dish. Add a layer of grated cheese mixed with chopped onion. Finally, sprinkle on the herbs.

Repeat the layer two more times or until all the ingredients are used, ending with spices.

3. Pour milk or stock over the dish. Sprinkle with seeds and bake at 350-400°F. for about 30 minutes, or until potatoes are tender and browned around the edges of the dish.

Tips

If you use a baking pan similar to one that you'd use for lasagna, your cooking time will be less and more of the exposed surface will have a chance to brown.

Oil the pan before cutting any vegetables.

Variation

Serve with fresh sprouts or grated carrots sprinkled on top.

*Raw potatoes tend to darken so assemble and bake at the same time.

Potato Kugel with Cheese

In Jewish culinary terms, kugel means pudding. This is a variation of that traditional Jewish dish.

Utensils

Grater for carrots and cheese
Cutting board or knife
Large bowl
Shallow casserole dish (approx. 10" x 10")

Ingredients

1. 1 cup grated natural cheese (3-4 oz.)
1 cup grated carrots (2 small)

2. 5 potatoes (about $1^1/_4$ lb.), scrubbed and chopped
1 garlic clove, peeled and minced
1 small onion, peeled and chopped
Water or stock

3. Herbs and spices to taste: thyme, parsley, dill
1-2 T. sesame seeds

4. Grated radishes or fresh alfalfa sprouts or fresh parsley

Directions

1. Place the grated cheese and carrots in large bowl and set it aside.

2. Puree the potatoes, garlic, and onion in a blender with a small amount of water or stock to get blender going. Mix with cheese and vegetables in the bowl.

3. Stir herbs into the mixture and pour into the oiled casserole.

Sprinkle the seeds and bake for about 45 minutes in a 350°F. oven, or until the edges are brown and the center of the dish is slightly firm.

4. Right before serving, garnish the dish with radishes, sprouts or parsley.

Tips

To reduce any discoloration of the potatoes, grate the cheese and carrots before cutting the potatoes. Oil the casserole with lecithin and safflower oil to eliminate sticking.

Special Potato Salad

What makes this dish special is that no mayonnaise is used. If you add fresh sprouts, it becomes extra special.

Utensils

Cutting board and knife
Blender or Jar with lid
Steamer
Platter for serving salad

Ingredients

1. Salad: 2 lbs. new potatoes, scrubbed well and left unpeeled

2. Minced fresh parsley
1-2 scallions, cleaned and chopped
$^1/_2$ red bell pepper, diced

3. Dressing: $^1/_2$ cup sesame, safflower or sunflower oil $^1/_4$ cup lemon juice
1-2 garlic cloves, peeled and minced
Dash of natural soy sauce (optional)

4. Topping: Alfalfa sprouts or cucumber slices
1-2 T. sesame seeds

Directions

1. Dice potatoes and steam until tender, but still firm. (Less than $^1/_2$ hour.) Allow to cool.

2. While the potatoes are cooking, prepare the vegetables. Mix and set them aside in a large bowl.

3. Buzz the dressing ingredients in a blender or shake them well in a jar. Refrigerate.

Toss the diced, cooled potatoes with the minced vegetables.

Add the dressing and toss.

4. Spoon the potato salad onto an attractive platter, leaving a "gutter" around the edges. Fill the gutter with alfalfa sprouts or wedges of cucumber.

Sprinkle with seeds and serve.

Tips

Dice the potatoes to reduce your cooking time.

Make the dressing ahead of time and refrigerate. (Flavors will have a chance to mingle.)

Variation

Add or use other vegetables such as zucchini or cucumber in the salad. Use other seeds such as poppy or caraway.

Spud Stew

This economical dish is perfect for cold winter nights when no one wants to fuss, but everyone wants a hearty meal.

Utensils

Large pot for stew
Measuring cup
Cutting board and knife
Attractive heatproof bowl or a soup tureen (optional)

Ingredients

1. 3 cups water or stock
1 cup dry lentils, soaked several hours (yield: about 2 cups)
3-4 medium potatoes, scrubbed and diced (about 1-1 $^1/_2$ lbs.)
1-2 small onions, peeled and chopped
1-2 celery stalks, scrubbed and chopped coarsely
2-3 carrots, scrubbed and sliced thinly or in small chunks
Herbs and spices to taste: garlic, natural soy sauce, thyme

2. 1-2 cups garden peas, fresh or frozen

Directions

1. Put all of the vegetables and seasonings in a large pot or dutch oven.

Cover and simmer until the potatoes are tender, but not mushy for about 35-45 minutes. (Add more water if you wish a soupier stew.)

2. During the last 5-10 minutes, stir in the peas. When you are ready to serve, transfer to a soup tureen or attractive casserole, if you .wish.

Tips

Soak the lentils for several hours or even overnight to reduce your cooking time.

If you have a crock pot, try It and ovoid using a pot and a casserole.

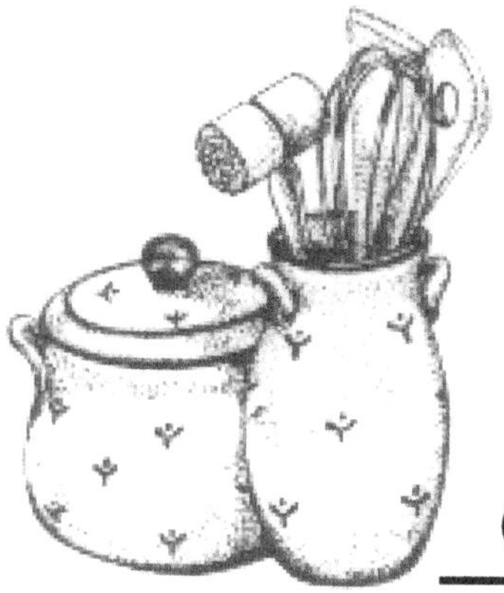

GRAINS & BEANS

Since all the dishes in this section use grains or beans, check Cooking Hints for general directions on how to cook these items. When a special grain is used, like cous-cous, the recipe will include special cooking instructions.

Note: Natural, unrefined, brown rice and other whole grains are more wholesome and nutritious than highly refined grains: the outer shell has not been milled.* Also, while soybeans are considered the best source of protein from the vegetable kingdom, other beans such as pinto, navy, and garbanzo can be substituted for maximum variety in your dishes. All are good protein sources.

*Pearled barley and cous-cous are more refined and should be used less frequently than the other grains.

Simple Stir Fries over Rice

This dish is not only colorful and tasty but fun to make, especially if you own a wok.

Utensils

Large saucepan for rice
Wok or large fry pan
Stirring spoon
Cutting board and knife

Ingredients

1. 2 cups uncooked brown rice
   4 cups water or stock
2. Sesame oil or stock for wok
   1 garlic clove, peeled and minced
   Broccoli stalks, scrubbed, peeled, and sliced thinly, crosswise into rings
   1-2 bell peppers, preferably red, washed and cut into slivers
   4-5 green onions (scallions), cleaned and chopped
   1-2 cups mung bean sprouts
   Additional stock or water if necessary

Directions

1. Cook the rice according to directions (see Cooking Hints).

2. When the rice is about done, clean and slice the vegetables. Preheat the wok and add a small amount of oil or stock.

Cook minced garlic for 1-2 minutes. Then add each of the ingredients in the order given, allowing 2-3 minutes of stir-frying between items. Add spices.

Add more stock (or water) if necessary to prevent sticking.

Spoon cooked rice onto platter and top with vegetables.

Tips

Start rice about 35 minutes before preparing vegetables.

Variation

Add almonds or cashews for crunchy vegetables.

Caraway Cabbage Stew

This hearty winter dish can be served elegantly in a tureen, or simply in the cooking pot.

Utensils

Measuring cup
Saucepan for rice
Large pot for stew
Mixing spoon or paddle
Cutting board and knife
Attractive casserole dish or soup tureen (optional)
Grater (If you ore using cheese)

Ingredients

1. 1 garlic clove, peeled and minced
1 onion, peeled and sliced
Small amount of tomato juice or sauce

2. 1 medium cabbage, sliced thinly or chopped coarsely
2 qts. tomato sauce or homemade spaghetti sauce (see Lynn's Special Spaghetti Sauce Recipe)

3. 3 cups cooked brown rice ($1^1/_2$ cups uncooked*)
Spices and herbs to taste
$^1/_4$ - $^1/_2$ cup caraway seeds
Water (if necessary)

Directions

1. Simmer the garlic and onion in a small amount of liquid until the onion is soft.

2. Add the cabbage and sauce and cook over medium heat for about 20 minutes or until cabbage is tender, but not mushy.

3. Stir in the cooked rice, add seasonings and seeds, and simmer for a few minutes more to allow the rice to become warm and for flavors to mingle.

If you want a soupier stew, add water to desired consistency. Serve in a heatproof casserole or soup tureen.

Tips

Pre-cook the rice and refrigerate.
Cut the cabbage thinly to reduce your cooking time.

Variation

1. Add a sliced bell pepper, green beans or other vegetable of your choice.

2. Add one cup of grated natural cheese with spices or place cabbage stew in a flat casserole dish, sprinkle with cheese, top with a few more seeds and bake until cheese melts and dish is warmed through.

*If the rice is not pre-cooked, start cooking first before beginning the rest of the stew.

Barley/Bean Bowl

This is a thick, hearty one-dish meal, perfect for cold, winter nights.

Utensils

Large roasting pan with cover (use cookie sheet for cover if necessary)
Fry pan for vegetables
Cutting board and knife
Measuring cup
Heatproof casserole (optional)

Ingredients

1. 1 cup uncooked pearled barley
1 cup dried aduki beans or other bean of your choice, soaked overnight and drained (if using a small bean like the aduki, freezing step is unnecessary)
4 cups water or stock

2. Butter, oil, stock, or tomato juice
8-10 scallions, rinsed, trimmed, and minced
1 zucchini, scrubbed and sliced
2 bell peppers, preferably red, washed, and chopped (seeds are also okay) and/or thinly sliced carrots
1-2 garlic cloves, peeled and minced
1-2 T. herbs and spices to taste: thyme, marjoram, dill, natural soy sauce

3. 1-2 T. sesame seeds, raw or roasted

Directions

1. Place the barley in an ungreased roasting pan and dry roast for 10 minutes.
Add the soaked and drained beans plus water or stock. Cover and bake until all water is absorbed (about 55 minutes in a 350° oven), stirring occasionally.

2. When the barley is almost done, take a frying pan and simmer the vegetables in a liquid until they are soft. Stir in the seasonings right at the end.

3. Add the seasoned vegetables to the cooked barley. Mix them into the grains, sprinkle the seeds on, and serve.
If you wish, transfer to an attractive heatproof bowl and serve.

Tips

Cut the vegetables while the barley Is baking, but cook for only 5-10 minutes before the barley is done. The vegetables will still be worm and the casserole can be served as soon as the vegetables and grains are combined. In between, you can prepare the salad and set the table.

Green Soybean Succotash

Green soybeans, unlike their yellow soybean relative, need no presoaking. They are more like lima beans and give this succotash a protein boost.

Utensils

Saucepan for beans
Fry pan for vegetables
Grater for cheese (if you are using It)
Measuring cup
Attractive heatproof dish

Ingredients

1. 2 cups washed green soybeans
5-6 cups water or stock

2. 2-3 cups corn kernels, fresh or frozen

3. $^{1}/_{2}$-1 red bell pepper, minced
3-4 scallions, cleaned and chopped
1 garlic clove, peeled and minced
1 small onion, peeled and minced
Water, stock or tomato juice
Herbs and spices to taste: natural soy sauce, thyme, oregano

4. Sesame or dill seeds
1 cup grated natural cheese (optional)

Directions

1. Cook the soybeans on a medium high heat in liquid for about 45 minutes, or until all but about $^{1}/_{2}$ cup of liquid is left and the beans are soft, but not mushy.

2. Add the corn and cook for 15-20 minutes more.

3. Simmer-saute the cut vegetables in a small amount of liquid until soft, but not mushy. Add seasonings near the end.

4. Spoon the cooked beans and corn into an ungreased casserole. Stir in the cooked vegetables. Sprinkle with seeds and eat while warm.

If you wish, sprinkle the cheese on before adding the seeds and bake in 300°F. oven just until the cheese melts.

Tips

Since this dish con be eaten as soon as it is assembled, hove the table set and salad ready.

Vege-Bobs with Cous-Cous

This make-ahead dish will impress even the most particular palate. While it takes extra steps to prepare, the results are worth it.

Utensils

8" bamboo skewers (9—10), available in kitchen shops and some supermarkets
Roasting pan (lasagna pan works well), with cover
Cookie Sheet
Cutting board and knife
Large pot for grains
Serving platter (heatproof If possible)

Ingredients

1. Sauce (or marinade):
   1 cup safflower or sesame or olive oil
   1 T. natural soy sauce
   1 cup tomato sauce or flavored spaghetti sauce
   $1^1/_2$ cup water or stock
   Spices to taste: garlic, thyme, rosemary

2. 1 onion, peeled and cut lengthwise into wedges
   1 bell pepper (red if possible), washed and cut into bite-size pieces $^1/_2$ eggplant, scrubbed and cut into small chunks (with or without skins)
   10-12 small mushrooms, washed with a soft cloth and cut in half lengthwise
   1 zucchini, scrubbed and cut into bite-size chunks (Feel free to use other firm vegetables of your choice.)

3. 2 cups cous-cous
   4 cups water or stock
   1-2 cups heated sauce left from marinating the vegetables

Directions

1. Place all of these ingredients in the blender and buzz for a few seconds.

   Pour half in the bottom of the roasting pan and keep other half in the blender.

2. Use skewers to pierce the vegetables. Each skewer should hold two of each cut vegetable (e.g., onion, pepper, eggplant, mushroom, zucchini). Repeat. Leftover pieces can be pierced at random.

   Place the skewered vegetables in the roasting pan with half of the marinade already poured in. Pour on the other $^1/_2$ of marinade; cover, and refrigerate for several hours or overnight.

   Before baking vege-bobs, pour off marinade and save. Bake at 350°F. for 20 minutes, then on broil for 5 minutes or until the edges of the vegetables turn crisp.

3. While the vege-bobs are in the oven, boil the water or stock. Pour over cous-cous in the saucepan. Cover and let all the water be absorbed, 15-20 minutes.

   Place cous-cous on large platter and put vege-bobs on it in spoke effect. Pour the extra sauce on and serve hot.

Tips

Prepare the vege-bobs the evening before you wish to eat them. Then Just pop them In the oven for 20-25 minutes before dinner. Warm the serving platter In the oven before baking the Vege-Bobs.

Variation

Short cut method: Skewer vegetables and heat marinade. Broil vegetables on skewers, pour on sauce and serve.

Calico Stuffed Peppers

Think of each stuffed pepper as a personal-sized casserole (i.e. the grains and vegetables as the filling and the pepper shells as the container or "dish" for every serving).

Utensils

Saucepan for peppers
Saucepan or roosting pan for millet
Fry pan for vegetables
Cutting board and knife
Casserole dish (optional)

Ingredients

1. 1 cup millet
4 cups water or stock

2. 6 flat-bottomed bell peppers, washed, tops and seeds removed. (Seeds can be added to vegetables.)

3. $1^1/_2$ cups diced vegetables of your choice: celery, carrots, onion, pepper, zucchini, yellow squash
Water, stock, or tomato juice
Herbs and spices to taste: Natural soy sauce, thyme, garlic

4. Seeds: dill, sesame or ground nuts: almond, pecans, cashews

Directions

1. Cook as you would rice on top of the stove; or prepare like barley in the oven. (See Barley/Bean Bake, p. 31)

2. When you are done, add the cooked vegetables from step 2.

3. While the millet is cooking, steam or par-boil peppers (not too soft). Place in a roasting pan with a small amount of water or stock or tomato juice on the bottom.

When the millet is almost done, cut and simmer-saute the vegetables in a small amount of water, stock, or tomato juice until the vegetables are soft but not mushy.

Add seasonings near the end and additional liquid if necessary to prevent burning.

When the vegetables are done, stir them into the cooked millet and then spoon into par-boiled peppers.

4. Sprinkle with nuts or seeds of your choice and bake in a 350°F. oven for a few minutes more, just to heat everything together.

Tips

For quicker reheating, cut stuffed peppers in half lengthwise; place In oven and bake until warmed through.

Variations

1. Spoon on tomato sauce and cheese, and top with seeds.

2. For a crunchy contrast, finely mince all the vegetables and add them raw to the cooked grains.

Bulghur Boats

This colorful, tasty and nutritious dish is perfect for fall meals, especially Thanksgiving, when acorn squash is readily available.

Utensils

Roasting pan
Pot or heatproof bowl for grains
Cutting board and knife
Attractive platter (heatproof)

Ingredients

1. 3 small acorn squash Water

2. 2 cups bulghur (toasted cracked wheat)
$3^1/_2$-4 cups water or stock (use a smaller amount for dryer grain)

3. 1 cup minced vegetables: garlic, onion, pepper, celery, yellow squash, Jerusalem artichoke
Herbs and spices: natural soy sauce, thyme, rosemary

4. Sesame seeds
Grated cheese (if you are using it)

Directions

1. Cut the squash in half (lengthwise). Scoop out the seeds and membrane. Place them face down in the roasting pan with 1″-2″ water. Bake until soft (about 45 minutes).

2. While the squash is in the oven, boil the water. Pour water over the grains placed in pot or bowl. Cover and let all water be absorbed (15-20 minutes).

3. While the squash and grains are "in the works," simmer-saute the minced vegetables until soft but not mushy. Add seasonings. Stir the seasoned vegetables into finished bulghur.

4. Top each stuffed squash with seeds or cheese and seeds, and bake until all is warmed through and the cheese melts.

Tips

Preheat the oven to 350°F.
Preheat the serving platter so boats will stay warm on the table.

Fried Rices

This dish uses wild rice as well as brown rice, providing extra nutrition along with extra flavor.

Utensils

Wok or fry pan Cutting board or knife

Ingredients

1. 1 cup brown rice, rinsed
   $^1/_2$ cup wild rice, rinsed
   3 cups water or stock

2. 2 cups cleaned and minced veggies: garlic, peppers, onions, or seal-lions, celery, mushrooms, squash, mung bean sprouts (the latter need not be cut)
   Butter, stock, or water (1 or 2 Tablespoons)
   Herbs and spices: ginger, cumin, dill, natural soy sauce

Directions

1. Cook the rices together in boiling water (see Cooking Hints). Chill.

2. Preheat wok or fry pan for 1 minute. First add the liquid and then the vegetables. Cook until they are almost soft.

Add the chilled rices and stir-fry until heated through. Add more liquid to prevent sticking if necessary. Serve hot.

Tips

Make your rices the day before and allow them to be well-chilled.

Variation

Add coarsely chopped almonds or cashew pieces to rice and vegetables for a crunchier texture.

Garbanzo Gumbo

The garbanzos in this okra-thickened recipe add a delicious, nutty flavor to a colorful casserole.

Utensils

Measuring cup
Large dutch oven or similar stew pot
Cutting board and knife
Large saucepan for garbanzos

Ingredients

1. 3 cups (cooked) garbanzos (1 cup soaked)

2. Small amount of tomato sauce
1 garlic clove, peeled and minced
1 onion, peeled and chopped
1-2 stalks celery, scrubbed and chopped

3. 10 oz. frozen okra (or fresh)
1 cup eggplant, scrubbed and diced (with peel)
2 cups tomato sauce

4. Herbs and spices to taste

Directions

1. Cook the frozen chickpeas while preparing the rest of the dish.

2. While the chickpeas are cooking, simmer-saute the garlic, onion, and celery in a small amount of tomato sauce (or spaghetti sauce) for 1-2 minutes (use stew pot).

3. Reduce heat and add the okra, eggplant and 2 more cups of sauce.
Cover and cook over medium heat until the okra and eggplant are tender (10-15 minutes).

4. Finally, drain the chickpeas and add to the simmering vegetables along with seasonings. Cook 5 minutes longer and serve.

Tips

Soak, drain, and freeze the chickpeas (garbanzos) the night before you intend to cook the meal.

Polygrain Pilaf

This hearty, colorful dish combines three nutritious grains into one delicious casserole.

Utensils

Measuring cup
Large roasting pan with lid
Cutting board and knife
Saucepan
Steamer

Ingredients

1. $^1/_2$ cup brown rice
$^1/_2$ cup toasted buckwheat groats (kasha)
$^1/_2$ cup whole millet

2. 1 T. dehydrated onion flakes
1 t. dehydrated garlic flakes
$3^1/_2$ cups boiling water or stock

3. 1-2 carrots, scrubbed and sliced into thin rings
1-2 cups garden peas (frozen if no fresh peas are available)

4. Seasoning to taste 1 T. oil or butter

Directions

1. Spread the rinsed grains in your roasting pan. Heat in 350°F. oven for 5-7 minutes, until grains are dry.

2. Add the flakes to the liquid and then to the grains. Stir, cover, and bake until liquid is almost absorbed; about 25 minutes.

3. While the grains are cooking, steam carrots, adding peas a few minutes afterwards. Steam until tender, not mushy.

4. When the grains are almost dry, remove cover, add carrots, peas and seasonings, and bake 4-5 minutes longer.

Remove and dot with butter or stir in oil and serve.

Tips

For a large family, double the recipe—low cost, high nutrition.

Hints on Cooking Grains

Cooking Raw Brown Rice

Since natural brown rice is the backbone of many dishes, I often cook twice the amount necessary for a recipe and refrigerate or freeze the rest for a later meal. Because rice expands—2 cups raw makes 6 cups cooked—it is a good budget stretcher as well as a nutritious food. Make it often. I find this is the best method for cooking rice.

1. Measure rice.

2. Boil twice as much water as rice.

3. Stir in rice and bring water to a second boil.

4. Lower the heat to a simmer. Cover tightly. Cook until all the water is absorbed (about 45 minutes).

5. Do *not* mix well until all the water is absorbed. If the rice is still not tender, add hot water and simmer for a few minutes more.

Cooking Pearled Barley

Use the same method but increase the water to 5 cups for each cup of grain. (Whole barley is more nutritious than pearled, but is completely different in texture, taste, and preparation.)

Cooking Millet

Use same method but cook in 4 cups water for every cup of millet.

Preparing a Pilaf

For a crunchy grain dish called a pilaf:

1. Toast or roast grains in a shallow baking pan for a few minutes.

2. Add boiling water or stock and cover until all the water is absorbed.

This method makes a drier, nuttier grain, and can be used for rice, barley, kasha or millet. (Follow cooking directions for water/grain proportions.)

Hints on Cooking Dry Beans*

This soaking, freezing, cooking method cuts down cooking time considerably. Moreover, I often freeze a large batch of beans and remove them as I need them, cooking them while I prepare the rest of the casserole. If you don't own a pressure cooker, this is the quickest method.

1. Soak the beans in water overnight, covered. Make sure to use plenty of water because the beans expand.

2. Drain beans the next day. Place on a cookie sheet in your freezer, separating beans as much as possible.

3. When thoroughly frozen, cook them in boiling water for about 1/2 hour. (Large beans may take a little longer.)

4. Save water for stock. Place beans in refrigerator unless you plan to use them right away.

Note; If you add carrots, onions, and celery to the bean water, your stock will be more flavorful.

*Lentils, black-eyed peas, and green soy beans do not have to be soaked, although soaking lentils or black-eyed peas will reduce cooking time.

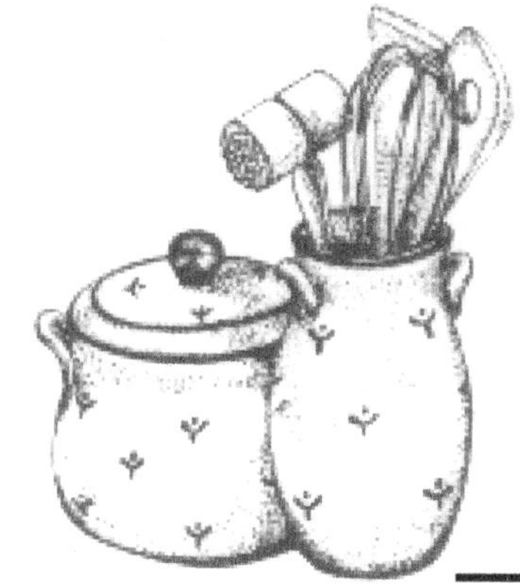

7 DAY MENU

For a complete reference on natural food definitions and products, I recommend Christopher Kilham's *Complete Shopper's Guide to Natural Foods,* a 176-page paperback published by Autumn Press, Brookline, Mass.

7 Day Menu

For meal planning, here are a few hints that might help you incorporate meatless casseroles into your daily menu:

1. Plan your menus visually as well as nutritionally; i.e. cook with color.
2. Try to use fruits and vegetables in season whenever possible.
3. Include raw foods in every meal.
4. Add lightly steamed vegetables to meals featuring heavily cooked dishes.
5. Aim for *one* main meal each day: The menus below can be used either for lunch or dinner.

Meal 1

Large salad of romaine lettuce, celery, alfalfa sprouts, seal-lions, and tomatoes (when in season).

Spaghetti Dorio (page 8) or
Spinach Spaghetti (page 9) or
Shells and Cheese (page 13)

Steamed zucchini with tomato sauce and/or bowl of soup.

Optional: Whole wheat garlic bread

Meal 2

Calico Coleslaw: red and green cabbage, celery chunks, and sunflower seeds

Potato Kugel (page 22) or
Sliced Potato Cheese Bake (page 21)

Steamed green beans with sesame seeds or slivered almonds

Meal 3

Small salad of spinach, tofu cubes, and scallions

Simple Stir Fries (page 26) over Brown Rice

Egg Drop or other Oriental or Asian-style soup

Meal 4

Salad with lettuce, scallions, sprouts and avocado

Caraway Cabbage Stew (page 27)

Whole wheat corn muffins

Meal 5

Bowl of alfalfa sprouts tossed with red onions and croutons

Chilled tomato soup (in summer) or hot tomato soup (in winter)

Garden Vegetables over Noodles (page 11)

Sesame bread sticks

Meal 6

Tossed salad using vegetables *not* in Vege-Bobs

Vege-Bobs over Cous-Cous (page 30)

Whole wheat pocket bread (pita)

Meal 7

Picnic, Buffet or Smorgasbord
Succotash (chilled in summer)

Chilled Pasta Platter (page 15) or
Spinach Spaghetti and Seeds (page 9) or
Confetti Macaroni Salad (page 17) or
Special Potato Salad (page 23) or

Celery, carrot, and cucumber spears
Hard boiled eggs or tofu cubes and
Cooked chickpeas sprinkled with herbs.

Recipes found in cookbook

GLOSSARY

Barley (whole hulled) - One of the oldest cultivated grains; when pearled, as is the usual form, the nutritious bran coating containing the B vitamins is lost.

Buckwheat - Not really a true grain like wheat since the fruit and not the seeds of the plant are eaten. It is used like a grain, however, and more commonly known as kasha when roasted.

Bulghur - A toasted cracked wheat that is very popular in Mid-East cookery—especially in the cold grain dish known as tabouli.

Cornmeal - Whole corn kernels milled into a coarse texture, but not germinated, overheated, or enriched with artificial nutrients; in other words, natural, whole germ cornmeal,

Cous-Cous - A grain as well as a dish made from hard durum wheat, but not considered a whole grain. When cooked, it is light and fluffy with a sweet grain taste.

Dutch oven - A large flat pot usually with a handle on either side or a thin metal handle like that found on a pail. Cast iron supposedly makes the best dutch oven dishes, but it is very heavy.

Fertile Eggs - Eggs from hens in which there is an active rooster in the yard. Generally, the feed is pure (no chemicals) and the chickens roam freely, laying their eggs at will.

Graham Flour - A whole wheat flour named after Sylvester Graham, an early leader in the field of dietary reform. There is usually more bran in this flour, giving it a coarser texture.

Grits - Refers to a smaller grind of grain than the whole grain, but not so fine as meal. For example, corn grits are larger pieces than corn meal.

Groats - Refers to the whole grain, such as buckwheat groats.

Hydrogenated - Usually refers to oils treated with hydrogen which change the molecular structure of oil in such a way that fat content is no longer digestible, and considered harmful by many nutrition-oriented doctors. Margarine is made solid through hydrogenation.

Jerusalem Artichoke - A member of the sunflower family, this tuber is supposed to be starch-free. When made into a flour and then incorporated into pasta, the resulting noodles are less starchy or pasty and look almost white.

Kelp - Type of seaweed often used as a salt or pepper substitute when dried and powdered; high in iodine.

Lecithin (liquid) - This is an extract usually taken from soybeans. It is used as an emulsifier (natural) and a preservative (natural) in confections, but works very well by itself or when combined with oil to coat bake pans. As a health benefit, it supposedly reduces cholesterol levels in the body.

Legume - A term used to designate the food categories of beans, peas and lentils; inexpensive form of protein as well as other nutrients such as calcium and iron, and a good source of fiber. Sometimes referred to as pulses.

Millet - A highly nutritious grain that can be used at breakfast, dinner, or ground into flour for baking needs. Good source of non-gluten grain for those on a gluten-free diet.

Miso - A seasoning paste made from aged and fermented soybeans, barley, or rice, plus sea salt and water. It adds a hearty flavor to dishes. Used originally in the Orient, but now a popular item in the western world as well.

Miso Cup™ - A trademark name of Edwards & Sons for powdered Miso that dissolves in hot water and can be easily used in soups, stews, casseroles, and dips. Like miso paste, it contains sea salt.

Nature Foods - General term used to describe foods that have not been refined and are still in their natural state, such as unsprayed peanuts, in unbleached shells. Natural peanut butter would be made without sugar or (artificial) additives, but made only of ground, unsprayed peanuts.

Oats - Generally thought of as oatmeal; in its whole form, called oatgroats which can be cooked as a cereal. The steel cut form also makes a coarse cereal. In the crushed or flaked form, it is used as a cooked cereal, in granola and familia, or as an ingredient in baking breads, cookies, or cakes. Considered to be high in nutrients (excepting the quick-cooking commercial oatmeal).

Organic Foods - Foods that have been grown on nutrient-balanced soil, free of pesticides or artificial soil enrichment.

Pilot - Literally a dish made with rice and meat; more liberal interpretation in vegetarian literature is toasting any grain in the oven, adding liquid, and baking until grains have absorbed all the liquid and are dry and nutty-tasting.

Polyunsaturated Oils - Refers to vegetable oils that are *not* saturated, that is, oils that can carry the fat soluble vitamins through the bloodstream as well as perform other important bodily functions that animal fats cannot. Most common types: corn, peanut, safflower, sunflower, and sesame oil. Even these should be used sparingly.

Rice - A popular grain in both white and brown, but only brown has the outer bran layer which contains valuable nutrients, especially the B vitamins. Try to obtain organically grown rice.

Rye Grains - Whole grains rich in nutrients, and sometimes tolerated by those allergic to wheat. Rye flour makes a tasty bread, but is usually mixed with whole wheat since rye makes a heavy bread.

Sauté - To fry quickly in a small amount of oil over high heat.

Semolina Flour - A white flour made by removing the bran and wheat germ from whole grain durum wheat. Used in pastas.

Simmer - To cook just below boiling point until liquid is reduced.

Simmer-Sauté - Two steps: very quickly fry vegetables in liquid, then reduce heat and let cook slowly.

Soy Sauce - A liquid extract made mainly from fermented soybeans. Also known as tamari. Commercial soy sauce is not a fermented product and generally contains a preservative.

Sprinkle - A trademark name for a powdered vegetable product that can be used as a salt substitute.

Sprouts - Seeds, beans and grains grown hydroponically (using water, not soil). When sprouted to maturity, 3-5 days, they can be eaten in salads, sandwiches, casseroles, etc.

Steamer - A colander-type utensil with legs; it is placed inside a pot of water but only the legs sit in the water. Vegetables are placed above the water and cooked by the steam. They are less soggy, crunchier, and more nutritious than when vegetables are boiled in water.

Stock or Broth - Liquid from cooking beans or vegetables in water. Often used as a basis for soups, stews, and casseroles.

Tamari - See soy sauce.

Tasty Tofu - A new product from Deep Roots Trading Co., in which whole herbs are added to the tofu.

Triticole - A hybrid grain obtained from crossing wheat with rye, but higher in essential amino acids (protein building blocks) than either wheat or rye. Used like wheat or rye in cooking, baking, or sprouting.

Tofu - Curdled soy bean milk made into a bland cheese-like consistency. Also known as bean curd. Originated in the Orient, but becoming more popular in America, especially because it is an easily-digested, less expensive source of high quality protein.

Whole grains - Grains with none of the vital nutrients removed, such as the outer coating (bran) and the germ of the kernel. Some of the more common ones are:

Whole Herb Seasoning - A mixture of healthful herbs and freeze-dried alfalfa sprouts. Formulated by Deep Roots Trading Company, Lewis-burg, PA, 17837.

Whole Wheat Berries - Another term for whole wheat grains containing the kernels or berries with bran and wheat germ intact. Can be cooked whole as cereal, but usually ground into flour for baking.

Wok - Cone-shaped Oriental utensil that sits on a rim above the heat. Vegetables are kept crunchy by stir frying in very little oil.

For a complete reference on natural food definitions and products, I recommend Christopher Kilham's Complete Shopper's Guide to Natural Foods; 176-page paperback published by Autumn Press, Brookline, MA, and costs.

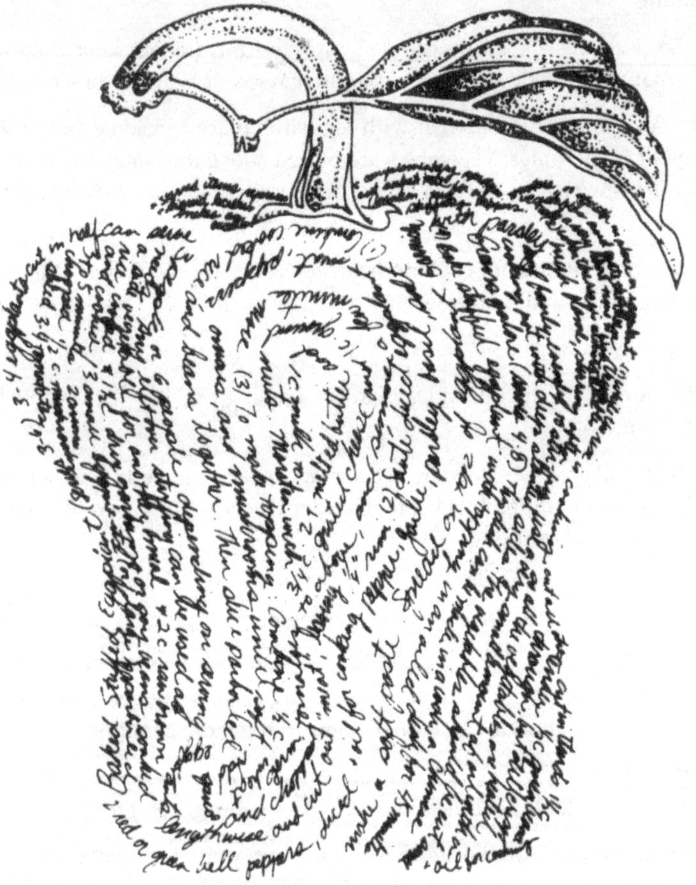